Hospitality and Assimilation

by Dirk J. Hart

AF826047

CRC Publications
Grand Rapids, Michigan

The author of this booklet, Dirk J. Hart, is minister of evangelism for Christian Reformed Home Missions, Grand Rapids, Michigan.

Unless otherwise indicated, Scripture quotations in this publication are from the HOLY BIBLE, NEW INTERNATIONAL VERSION, © 1973, 1978, 1984, International Bible Society. Used by permission of Zondervan Bible Publishers.

Healthy Church series. Hospitality and Assimilation, © 1992, 1999 by CRC Publications, 2850 Kalamazoo Ave. SE, Grand Rapids, MI 49560. All rights reserved. With the exception of brief excerpts for review purposes, no part of this book may be reproduced in any manner whatsoever without written permission from the publisher. Printed in the United States of America on recycled paper. ♻

We welcome your comments. Call 1-800-333-8300 or e-mail us at editors@crcpublications.org.

ISBN 1-56212-454-4

10 9 8 7 6 5 4 3 2 1

To evangelize is to declare and demonstrate the good news of the kingdom of God. Its goal is this: that people should be converted, become members of the church, and themselves become evangelizers. To accomplish this, new members should be welcomed and assimilated into the fellowship and mission of the church. For many churches, however, assimilation is the most difficult aspect of evangelism.

The Bible and Hospitality

The Bible teaches that hospitality is one of the marks of the people of God. A holy congregation, truly set apart for service to God, cannot be an elitist, exclusionary, or isolated congregation.

The Old Testament is clear on how God's people should treat strangers and foreigners:

> *When an alien lives with you in your land, do not mistreat him. The alien living with you must be treated as one of your native-born. Love him as yourself, for you were aliens in Egypt. I am the LORD your God (Lev. 19:33-34).*

The "cities of refuge" in ancient Israel—places where those involved in involuntary manslaughter could flee from revenge—were open to the aliens as well as to the Israelites (Num. 35:15). David goes so far as to identify himself and his people with aliens. In the assembly of God's people he prays, "We are aliens and strangers in your sight, as were all our forefathers" (1 Chron. 29:15; see also Ps. 39:12). He expresses thereby an utter dependence on God and a place of privilege in the heart of God, for God shows no partiality and loves the alien (Deut. 10:17-18). Foreigners are ranked with the widow and fatherless as those for whom God's people must have special concern (Jer. 7:6).

In the New Testament the mystery of the church is unfolded: Gentiles and Jews are "members together of one body, and sharers together in the promise in Christ Jesus" (Eph. 3:6). In Christ, therefore, there are no longer any foreigners and aliens. In the church, national origin and ethnic identity are superseded by unity in Christ. All are members of God's household (Eph. 2:19). At the same time, all are "aliens and strangers in the world" (1 Pet. 2:11). Nevertheless, in a social sense some remain strangers—people whom we don't know, who are different from us, or who do not belong to the church. The church is called upon to minister to these people. "I was a stranger and you invited me in," Jesus says (Matt. 25:35).

Hospitality is a hallmark of the Christian church. "Offer hospitality to one another without grumbling," writes Peter (1 Pet. 4:9). Paul says simply, "Practice hospitality" (Rom. 12:13). Biblical hospitality involves not only giving something, it often entails receiving unexpected blessings. The author to the Hebrews hints at this when he writes, "Do not forget to entertain strangers, for by so doing some people have entertained angels without knowing it" (Heb. 13:2). When Abraham received three strangers, he found himself entertaining the Lord himself and he received the promise of a son (Gen. 18:1-15). The travelers to Emmaus had a personal encounter with the risen Christ when they invited a stranger in for supper (Luke 24:13-32). Hospitality, the art of creating friendly space for the strangers, brings with it unexpected rewards.

Assimilation and the Early Church

Soon after the early church began in Jerusalem it encountered assimilation problems. Grecian Jews complained that "their widows were being overlooked in the daily distribution of food" (Acts 6:1). Immediately the apostles asked for the appointment of seven spiritually mature men to solve this problem. Today we call these people deacons—they might also be called the church's first membership assimilation or congregational life committee. Creating friendly space for people different from the majority requires an organized effort. Congregational hospitality must be planned and supervised.

The early church encountered other assimilation problems: How can the faith and fellowship circle be open to receive new people who are different from the main body of believers? Peter was helped to overcome his prejudice against Gentiles by means of a vision (Acts 10). The first Jerusalem synod dealt specifically with the problem of Gentiles and Jews as members of the same household of God. On that occasion James said, "We should not make it difficult for the Gentiles who are turning to God" (Acts 15:19).

Assimilation Problems in the Church Today

Such problems continue to plague the church to this day. Everyone knows of a church where the back door is wide open—new members join frequently, but almost as many leave because they never feel part of the body. In some churches, new members seldom join unless they are related to someone in the church—a stranger is rarely made to feel at home. In other churches visitors get a cold reception—or worse, are stared at and never spoken to. Still other churches convey the message, "You have to wear a three-piece suit to worship here," or "We don't have much of a nursery so families with small children should look elsewhere," or "We emphasize the family—single adults are not welcome."

Assimilation problems are complicated by the "homogenous unit principle": people prefer not to cross barriers of race, class, or language when they become Christian. This is not so much a theory or approach as it is an observation of what has happened throughout much of church history. It is true that churches do grow faster and encounter fewer problems when they reach people who are most like themselves.

To call this a guiding principle by which a church should live denies the biblical teaching on hospitality and the unity of the body of Christ. While churches will most likely grow along natural friendship and kinship lines, they must always show openness and hospitality to persons who are different, seeking to structure the church in such a way that these people will feel part of the fellowship. At the same time, Christians can rejoice in the variety of churches in which people of a particular language and culture seek to reach others like themselves.

The homogenous unit principle tells us that it is more difficult to assimilate "different" believers. Such people often drop out of a church not for lack of faith, but for lack of friends. They do not feel at home.

The Church Must Want to Grow

Hospitality and assimilation begin when churches want to grow. The entire congregation, especially the leaders, must have a missionary heart that rejoices whenever new members are added to the fellowship. Members see growth as essential for the church's well-being and a blessing for all. The desire to grow is the catalyst that enables a church to deliberately organize and structure for growth.

A church that wants to grow not only receives those people who ask to become members (and who meet the membership standards), but also deliberately invites new people to join. And it ensures that such people are ministered to and included in meaningful ways so that they gladly speak of the church as "our church."

Characteristics of Assimilated Members

A church can start to examine its hospitality by asking new members, "What are the characteristics of an assimilated member?" Ask this question of new members since longtime members may be assimilated for reasons that have long since disappeared. A new member, however, should be able to identify some specific reason why he or she has joined the church and intends to stay.

Following are some reasons why new members stay:

- **They are enthusiastic about their faith commitment, their congregation, and their pastor.** They will say things such as "This is a really friendly church," "The pastor is a good preacher," "My family feels at home here," "The youth group meets a real need for my teenagers."

- **They have a task or function in the church.** They have identified their spiritual gifts and have been assigned responsibilities in line with those gifts. New members should become active in ministry within six months. People who are otherwise noncommittal will become alive and enthusiastic if they're involved in a task. If new members don't become involved, they are likely to "sit and soak." Give them a task, and they will feel a vital part of what's going on. Whereas justification is by grace, says Lyle Schaller, assimilation is frequently by works. The members who in some way participate in the church's ministry identify with and "own" that ministry.
- **They have a warm and personal relationship with the pastor.** They feel the pastor is interested in them, knows them, and is prepared to serve them. Consequently, they willingly listen to sermons and follow pastoral leadership.
- **They are involved in a small group** that meets at least once, preferably twice, a month. The group's purpose may be fellowship, study, or service; it may be a sports activity or associated with a specific task. Small groups give new members the opportunity to know and be known in a way that is not possible in the larger worship setting. New members don't have to know everyone in the church in order to feel like they belong. They can find that sense of belonging in a small group of people they know well. The larger the congregation, the more crucial this requirement is.
- **They know at least six or seven people in the congregation whom they identify as friends.** New members who do not form such attach-

ments within six months of joining are usually on their way out the back door.

- **They feel their relationship to God is strengthened and nourished in the church.** This may be their initial reason for joining; but it will not be enough to keep them in the church if they do not develop friendships.

Ideally, all these characteristics should apply to all members, including long-term members. They are especially important to new members who have no relatives in the church, to those who have never been a member of that denomination, and to new Christians.

The Hospitable Church

The hospitable church also has certain characteristics that identify it as a church equipped to attract, receive, and assimilate new members.

- **Worship services are a high point of the congregation's life** and are conducted with sensitivity to visitors and new believers. Members gladly bring friends and neighbors to church. Guests are welcomed and identified. Ushers and greeters are trained. Sermons are positive, include a clear call to commitment, and articulate the good news. There is opportunity for socializing and refreshments before or after the worship service. Guests will hear from the church within a week by phone, letter, or personal visit.
- **The congregation has a well-defined concept of ministry** that includes an evangelistic strategy. The leaders and members are committed to the concept of ministry, and the evangelistic strategy has a strong follow-up program. The goals attached to the concept of ministry are measur-

able, success is celebrated, and new goals are set annually. Inquirers are introduced to the concept of ministry in the new member's class. Some churches may ask everyone to sign a "membership covenant" that spells out the church's expectations of its members and contains a summary of the concept of ministry.

- **The church has a new members class** that is attended by all who join the congregation, whether by transfer or profession of faith. The class is held at least twice a year.
- **The spiritual gifts of all members are identified,** with the expectation that members will use their gifts in church and kingdom service. Members with the gift of hospitality are active in the assimilation process. New members are regularly given assignments that fit their spiritual gifts. Be careful, however, not to pull them into just any kind of activity. New members are usually very willing to get involved—sometimes too willing. They may take on commitments that overtax their abilities or strain their willingness to help. Their first tasks should be simple, entry-level duties. As they become more confident and their gifts become more evident, they can take on new and more challenging tasks.
- **New members are expected to join in some group or activity that places them in contact at least once a month with other members.** The church cheerfully adds new groups several times a year in order to accommodate new members or, alternatively, divides the congregation into households or shepherding groups of some kind.
- **New members are assigned a sponsor** who will befriend them, help them feel at home in the church, and introduce them to other members.

- **There is a public welcome for all who join the church.** Usually this is done in a morning worship service. If this is done twice a year, the public welcome is associated with a reception after the morning service or with a potluck supper on Saturday evening.
- **The church has a hospitality committee, a new members committee,** or a congregational life committee that plans and monitors the assimilation of each new member for one year and alerts the pastor or elders when a new member shows signs of losing interest.
- **Key leadership positions in the church are open to qualified new members.** In churches that come from a single ethnic background, new members may find it difficult to be accepted into leadership positions, even though they are highly qualified. The subtle message they receive is, "You're welcome to belong to our church, but since you don't share a common background we can't trust you with leadership." As a result, new members will want to look for a church where they're accepted and respected.

  If, on the other hand, a church opens its leadership to qualified new members—whatever their background—it says to all new members, "This is truly your church. We trust you. We value your contribution. We want you to help shape the direction of our life together."

Few churches will have all of these characteristics. But the church that takes hospitality seriously and wants to grow will have at least six of the nine fully functioning.

What Church Leaders Should Know

- **New members are valuable assets.** They bring new energy to the church. New members are eager to see the church be vital and strong. Each one brings a spiritual gift for upbuilding the church or for outreach. They also come with an optimistic view of the church's future.

  New members will have a strong loyalty to your congregation. They've chosen your church because it meets their needs; they want to be a part of you. They like the programs and the pastor; if they didn't, they wouldn't have joined your church. New members also bring a fresh perspective. Those who come from other churches may bring spiritual understanding, better ways of doing things, and skills learned in other settings. New Christians also have an extensive circle of non-Christian friends and acquaintances to reach for Christ.

- **Most churches need improvement in hospitality and assimilation.** Most of us are convinced our churches are friendly. And we are—to our own members and to relatives and friends who visit. That's only natural since there is already a connection. But when people come with no ready-made connections, the story is often different.

  Growth in hospitality and assimilation usually begins with honest self-assessment. As you evaluate your church's hospitality, be open to the comments of those who visited and didn't return, of new members, and of former members. Changing old patterns isn't easy, but it's possible. It takes intentional planning and new training. It means recruiting the right people and keeping track of what's happening to new members. And it's worth the effort.

- **Assimilating your young people is crucial.** Don't focus your efforts only on people coming in from the outside. It's just as important to help existing members feel more a part of the church. The young people in your church especially need your encouragement and help in becoming vitally involved in the church's ministry. If the youth aren't encouraged to find their spiritual gifts and to use them in the church, they often drop out and expend their energies elsewhere.

  This holds true for inactive or fringe members of the church as well. Those on the periphery need a sense of belonging, a sense that they are contributing something valuable to the church's life. Inactivity is a sign that departure may be near. Such members need to be reengaged through friendship, participation in small groups, or involvement in a ministry.

- **People join a friendly church.** In fact, friendliness is often the most important factor in a person's decision to join a church—rating above attractive facilities, good location, excellent programs, and good preaching. Why is friendliness so important? Because people want to be wanted. We want to be noticed, to have friends who enjoy our company. When we come to a place where no one seems to notice or to reach out in friendship, we get the message that we aren't wanted—and we usually won't return. Those who value warmth in relationships desire to be a part of a church where such relationships are present.

- **Assimilation is a key link between evangelism and church growth.** Church members may do a wonderful job of evangelizing their friends and neighbors, but the church won't grow unless it assimilates those new believers into its life.

Converts who remain on the fringe of the church's life will find other places to worship; or, worse, they may leave their newfound faith.

Every believer needs to be a member of Christ's body, the church, and to be connected to other members in fellowship. If a church is unprepared to enfold new believers into its life and ministry, it cuts these new Christians off from the nurture so greatly needed in the first stages of their faith. Churches that are prepared to receive new converts will be the most likely to grow through evangelism.

- **Leadershp is crucial.** Pastors, elders, and deacons must not only hold out the vision of an outreaching church but also model this vision. The friendliness of the church usually reflects the friendliness of its leaders. For this reason, the pastor and council members should be in the church foyer before the worship service to greet guests and members. After the service, council members should take the initiative to reach out to guests, engaging them in conversation and introducing them to other members.

Check Your Ratios

A church that wants to attract and incorporate new people needs to have its ratios in order. Research by the Institute of American Church Growth Data Bank indicates that the following minimum ratios are essential for a church that is serious about evangelization and incorporation.

- **Role/Task Ratio.** At least sixty roles and tasks should be available for every hundred members in your church. Any fewer than this creates an environment that produces inactive members.

Make your new roles and tasks focused on meeting needs and changing lives.

- **Small Group Ratio.** There should be at least seven small groups in your church for every hundred members. If there are too few small groups in which members can build meaningful relationships, a large number of inactive people will exit through the back door. Effective small group life is fundamental to growth and incorporation.
- **New Small Groups Ratio.** Of the small groups that now exist in your church, one of every five should have been started in the last two years. Groups tend to reach a saturation point somewhere between nine to eighteen months after their formation and will, in most cases, no longer effectively assimilate new people. The remedy is new groups that involve new converts and members.
- **Friendship Ratio.** Each new convert or member should be able to identify at least seven new friends in the church within the first six months. This is a crucial time factor since new members not integrated into the body within that time period will usually drop out.
- **Visitor Ratio.** Of the first-time visitors who live in the church's ministry area, three of every ten should be actively involved within a year. Studies indicate that churches with an effective strategy can expect to see four of every ten local visitors return. An incorporation strategy that focuses specifically on these second-time visitors will result in 70-75 percent joining within a year.
- **Board Ratio.** One of every five council members should have joined the church within the last

two years. New members are open to new ideas and direction, and their presence on the council assures all new members that the decision-making structure of the church is open to them.

- **Staff Ratio.** The church should have one full-time staff member for every 150 persons in worship. If the ratio reaches 1 to 250, it is unusual to see any significant increase in active membership. While more persons may join the church, the back door will open wider and wider (from *Institute of American Church Growth Newsletter,* 1984).

Dr. D. James Kennedy defines successful witnessing as "sharing the gospel in the power of the Holy Spirit and leaving the results to God." The hospitable church will want to change this definition to "sharing the gospel in the power of the Holy Spirit and *expecting* the results from God." Such churches will then demonstrate that expectation by making room for new members in the fellowship, service, and leadership of the church.

Recommended Resources

Dykema, Earl D. *Focus Your Ministry.* Grand Rapids, Mich.: CRC Publications, 1999.

Schaller, Lyle E. *Assimilating New Members.* Nashville, Tenn.: Abingdon, 1978.

Small Groups That Work. Grand Rapids, Mich.: CRC Publications, 1988.

Stam, Jeff. *Welcome and Enfold.* Grand Rapids, Mich.: CRC Publications, 1999.

Stark, David. *Seven Steps to Successful Small Group Ministry; Design and Launch a Successful Small Group; Step by Step Small Group Leader Training; Learning Together; Working Together; Being Together; Caring Together.* St. Paul, Minn.: Church Innovations, 1995.

VanderGriend, Alvin J. *Discover Your Gifts and Learn How to Use Them.* Grand Rapids, Mich.: CRC Publications, 1997.

Vander Zee, Ruth. *Discover Your Gifts and Learn How to Use Them, Youth Version.* Grand Rapids, Mich.: CRC Publications, 1998.

Warren, Rick. *The Purpose Driven Church.* Grand Rapids, Mich.: Zondervan, 1995.

Small groups are a vital component of any assimilation strategy. Small Group Ministry Representatives throughout Canada and the United States are available to conduct workshops, provide consulting, and answer your small group questions. For the name of the Small Group Ministry Representative nearest you, call toll-free 1-800-266-2175.